The Myths on Exercise

The Myths on Exercise

Michael Evans

To order additional copies of this book, contact:
Xlibris
1-888-795-4274
www.Xlibris.com
Orders@Xlibris.com
770878

Contents

To preface this article let me start out by saying that no 1 rule is the same for everyone.

Every person is an individual and needs to learn their own body's signals that exercise may be too much or too little.

I am also NOT a doctor and make no claims medically.

You should know when it comes to your health Medicine and Doctors have their place….it just is not always the first place and many time the last place.

Also if you have already had surgeries (i.e. neck or spine surgeries, pins, screws, prosthetics, pace makers or any other foreign material in your body.) You will need to take extra precautions while exercising.

Once the mechanics of the human body has been altered it can no longer function "completely "as it was intended to.

However this does not mean it's ok to park yourself on a couch and never do anything about your fitness level.

Fitness is not about vanity, your body was never intended to be dormant.

It needs to move to survive.

So your question: **Who am I to tell you that you don't have to listen to your doctor?**

Who I am is a person who after having doctors tell me I was to wind up in a wheelchair in my early 40's due to a "rare muscle disorder", (Charcot-**Marie-Tooth** disease (CMT) is an inherited disorder of **progressive** peripheral nerve dysfunction resulting in numbness and weakness. ... The same disease was described by Howard Henry **Tooth** in his Cambridge dissertation in 1886 under the name of **peroneal progressive** muscular atrophy.)....decided to break free of the main stream medical opinions and take my health into my own hands.

It was not an easy task because up until this very moment everything I knew in life to be true was "Trust your Doctor" and I may have if he had given me some sort of options, possibilities, Hope. Why wouldn't you tell me maybe I should eat better, drink more water, stop drinking soda pop or for the love of God, eat some vegetables!!

Instead I got a life sentence.

Daily life for me was a constant struggle, and although I had become accustomed to the pain and discomfort I had many things other people take for granted (like getting up off the floor) where a task for me.

At the the time I was living it I never really thought about it…..The daily issues I had where "normal life" for me. **No one gave me the option to feel better so how could I know.**

The truth is no one will ever give you an option to feel better because you being sick and on pills is big business. If you want to feel better its on you to find out what works for you.

Question the answers and look for better options.

I trusted my doctors to help me. Don't make that mistake ever. Be in charge of your own body and health.

Now you must understand I was in my early 20's when I got the news about this disorder I have.

When you are in your early 20's and someone says this will happen to you in your early 40's, your 20 year old brain say to you "that's like a million years from now", so what did I do with the information I got back then.....nothing.

It wasn't till many years later around age 37 that it hit me like a truck.

At that time in my life I was an executive for a major company, working ridiculous hours, getting little sleep, traveling all over and eating the worst food possible for anyone let alone someone with a muscle disorder.

So one Saturday afternoon, while watching a Yankee baseball and eating a bag of potato chips....I ran out of chips....ofcourse needing more chips to finish watching the game, I tried to stand up.

My wife at the time had to lend me a hand and pick me up off the couch.

Reality has reared its ugly head.

Wheelchair is all I could think.

So I started with what I knew…..ask Doctor Google.

"How do I keep my fat ass out of a wheel chair" "Oh and by the way I have CMT"

Doctor Googles answer? 18 million responses of which maybe 2 actually had good information. But hey…It was a start down the road of health and fitness.

Health 101:

1. Drink More Water, and when you think you have had enough for the day….drink more.

Being properly hydrated helps you.

2. Stop eating food that isn't food.

Boxed, canned, processed food like substances full of ingredients you can't pronounce are only killing you faster than time will. Add to that any disorders you may have and these fake foods are multiplying their symptoms by the millions.

Organic foods (for the most part) are foods in their natural unaltered state and are what your body needs to run as Mother Nature intended (Nutrient dense food).

3. Exercise consistently.

Cardiovascular exercise simply rushes two KEY things to all parts of the body that promote healing and health.

Blood and Oxygen.

Not to mention many other lifesaving effects such as,

Decreased resting heart rate.

Increased stroke volume at rest. (Heart works less and pumps more blood).

Improved circulation

Blood pressure can decrease by 10 mmhg

Blood volume increases

Weight lifting presents a whole other list of amazing health benefits.

Strength training increases **bone density**,

Builds a stronger heart,

Reduces your resting blood pressure,

Improves blood flow, halts muscle loss,

Helps control blood sugar,

Improves cholesterol levels, improves your balance and coordination

No before you panic because your doctor put you on "restrictions", remember what we have already discussed.

No one is completely broken. Start where you can, at the ability you currently have and get stronger one day at a time. It's what the body is intended to do.

The one thing to always remember on your fitness journey is, this is not a race, and it will not be fast.

So relax and enjoy the process.

Do what you can until you can do more.

Strive to be better at a pace your body can tolerate, (and you are the boss on this).

Reminder as you read along: Surgeries and other outside interventions

Once the mechanics of the human body has been altered it can no longer function "completely "as it was intended to.

Work within your ability until you can do more.

There is way more to learn but this is the start for anyone currently drinking a Code Red while reading this.

These 3 SIMPLE fundamental changes with set your body back on a track to repair itself as it was intended to do.

I can't say this enough….Just because you may be sick or injured or have a "disorder or handicap" now, doesn't make it a life sentence.

I decided I was NOT going to be in a wheel chair and I put my mind to it.

That's not where the story ends.

After seeing the infomercial for P90x about 9 million times on TV, I bought it thinking no worries, easy right? WRONG!

Oh yeah did I mention I was a smoker back then also?

P90x damn near killed me. However what I did learn is the art of "modifying".

Take a workout routine and fit it to your current abilities and it can grow as you do.

So I did a few days of P90x trying to keep up with the oiled down, beautifully ripped athletes they had on the video and I quickly realized no amount of oil was gonna help my sorry ass keep up with them.

So I humbled myself and stepped back to my ability. Take note of that last sentence. If you truly want to succeed in your fitness journey, check your EGO at the door. The only race happening here is you against you….. Be better tomorrow than today and make that a habit.

So I started over at the ability I had.

I showed up every day and did the workouts, even though my body was in pain from the prior days workout.

I took the rest days they said to take and I did the workouts when they said to workout.

I cleaned up my diet to the best of my knowledge at that time (as I was still learning to break old habits).

I took measurements and photos before I started and during the process and still today.

You need these things so you can look back and see for your own eyes your progress because on a day to day basis you will not see it and you can get frustrated.

Progress pics and measurements are a key ingredient to success.

My body, my life, my responsibility.

Far too often I see people who have been given a restriction by their doctor, for instance to NOT lift anything over 20 lbs. due to a "back problem"

Then you see the same people lift up their 5 year old to hug them…..well if you ask me, if your 5 year old is under 20lbs…that's a whole other topic of issues.

So why is it ok to lift some things and not others? Simply because one is called "Exercise'?

Why is exercise so demonized?

It's one of the most import things in your life and second only too proper nutrition.

Seeing other people struggle with "disabilities "and know what I learned the hard way myself is what made me decide to become a personal trainer myself.

So after getting my certifications, I started teaching others how to take back their lives.

Limited mobility doesn't mean you can't exercise

When you exercise, your body releases endorphins that energize your mood, relieve stress, boost your self-esteem, and trigger an overall sense of well-being. If you're a regular exerciser currently sidelined with an injury, you've probably noticed how inactivity has caused your mood and energy levels to sink. This is understandable: exercise has such a powerful effect on mood it can treat mild to moderate depression as effectively as antidepressant medication. However, an injury doesn't mean your mental and emotional health is doomed to decline. While some injuries respond best to total rest, most simply require you to reevaluate your exercise routine with help from your doctor or physical therapist. If you have a disability, severe weight problem, chronic breathing condition, diabetes, arthritis, or other ongoing illness you may think that your health problems make it impossible for you to exercise effectively, if at all. Or perhaps you've become frail with age and are worried about falling or injuring yourself if you try to exercise. The truth is, regardless of your age, current physical condition, and whether you've exercised in the past or not, there are plenty of ways to overcome your mobility issues and reap the physical, mental, and emotional rewards of exercise.

Lets talk your Health and Fitness

Do you care?

That's step one....here is why you should

The health problems associated with lack of exercise and or obesity are numerous. Obesity is not just a cosmetic problem. It's a health hazard. Someone who is 40% overweight is twice as likely to die prematurely as is an average-weight person and add disabilities on top of this it only gets worse. This is because obesity has been linked to several serious medical conditions, including:

Myself AND Doctors generally agree that the more obese a person is the more likely he or she is to have health problems. **People who are 20% or more overweight can gain significant health benefits from losing weight.** This is just for someone without the added disability issues.

Now for all the Excuses

1. I don't have the time (REALLY cause you sure had time to watch the football game and eat nachos and bean dip didn't you)

2. I don't have the energy to exercise.....Ok vicious circle here.....get your ass off the couch and exercise and you will get the energy you need to get it done.

3. I won't eat "diet food". Get educated before you make statements like this. Food that is good for you does not taste bad....unless you eat doormats for fiber....who does that? I suggest a good Nutritionist for proper food recommendations.

4. Here is the one that totally just torques me beyond belief.

"I only eat one time a day, why don't I lose any weight?"

Ummm...maybe because you're starving yourself and your metabolism has shut down. Not to mention the multitude of other issues you are causing yourself. You need to eat 5 to 6 small meals a day along with exercise to fix this.

I could go on with the list of excuses I have been given but I think you get the point....an excuse is only that...an excuse

You have the power to do anything you want (even if it's just small)....you only need the want and desire to make it happen. Far too many times the individual defeats themselves without trying...or they try for a short amount of time and give up....Please please do not do this to yourself....your size and age do not matter....you can change anytime you are ready for the journey....the human mind, body and spirit are the most amazing machines. Taken care of properly they can run and run hard for many many years!

Michael Jordan once said "I've failed over and over and over again in my life and that is why I succeed."

Learn to love your failures as each time you do you learn how to succeed.

Again remember to stress less about working out. Relax. Whether you work out in the gym or home, just do it, something, just get started. Force yourself to just get some time in. Every day you do its gets easier to exercise. Not that the exercise should be easy, just you're more likely to want to.

Getting your mind right

As well as the physical challenges you face, you may also experience emotional struggles pondering exercising. It's common for people to get in their own heads about their health constraints and want to avoid working out at home or anywhere else.

Don't focus on your health issue. Focus only on the things you can do and forget the rest.

The more physical challenged you are, the more innovative you will need to get to locate an exercise program that works for you. If you used to jog or cycle, but injury, disability, or illness makes them no longer options, you may need to try new exercises. With some trial and error, it's very likely that you'll find something you can do just as much.

Be proud when you make the effort to exercise, even if it's not very successful at first. It will get easier the more you practice.

I can't stress enough the importance of letting go of old habits. The bad ones that have gotten you nowhere. You know the saying "if you always do what you always did you always get what you always got". Which is fine if you got all you want from it but if not it's time to change it up.

What do you want to do, what do you want to be? Set that goal in your head. Write it down if you need to but get your mind wrapped around it. There is no pill or quick fix, only persistence and dedication to you and where you want to be. Goals people. You have to have them. Otherwise you're just a human tree growing root.

Largely you are going to be dealing in your head with all you have been taught by the medical society.

Years and years of "take this pill".

I've learned that either you control your attitude or it controls you. That we are responsible for what we do, no matter how we feel. Heroes are the people who do what has to be done when it needs to be done. Circumstances may have influenced who you are, but YOU are responsible for who you become.

Make your life how you want it. It's ...ALWAYS up to you!

However, there are extenuating circumstances that may dictate seeking the advice of your doctor.

As stated before everyone is different and the only thing that truly needs to happen is you need to be involved in how your body functions and Intune to how you feel.

The human body has tons of signals it sends out to tell you its current condition.

This may sound complicated and some truly can be but when it comes to exercise, your body will make it WELL known when it is time to back off or be done for the day.

In order for you to achieve a fitness level you are happy with it comes down to being completely honest with yourself. You have to become your own "Personal Trainer".

Tell yourself when to take it easy, then yell at yourself when you are just being lazy.

There are 2 major issues with getting back into shape especially if dealing with disabilities.

1. Support from those around you. You need positive support or none at all…no negativity allowed.

2. Taking the stress of it all off your mind. (Society. Well lazy people really, put such a stigma on fitness and health).

If you're not one of those people who can just jump right in and go go go then ease into it. Let your mind wrap itself around the concept. Watch the infomercials on fitness. Go to the gym and just watch what goes on. Do what you need to take the fear out of it.

You have to remember, this is a marathon of fitness and life. Not a sprint.

It took years to get out of shape, what a few more months or years to get back into shape.

For some this may mean just getting off the couch and walking a few hundred steps down to the corner and back, a few more minutes sweeping the floors or deciding to use the push mower instead of the rider.

Here is an idea....instead of driving around for 20 minutes waiting for a parking spot right next to the supermarket door, try earning your dinner and parking out a ways in the lot and walking. I know its an outrageous concept, but try it.

You will be surprised how if you just start. Get up and do something how much better you will start to feel.

The human body was designed to move and be tested. It will grow and repair itself as you move it.

Short of growing a limb back the human body has an amazing system capable of fixing almost anything!

Here is the trick. You have support that system with proper nutrition and exercise.

Think about is this way. How many times have you been out for a drive in the county and as you dive along you see old car after old car out in the middle of a field with weeds and trees growing out of it.

Totally broken down and rusted.

Well that car didn't get there by accident. It was shiny and new once and it got in that field because it moved and someone drove it there.

But as time passed and it didn't move....nature took over and is now working on recycling it back to the earth.

Well park your butt in a chair for too long and nature will do the exact same thing to you.

It doesn't matter what disability you may have (remember the no one rule applies to everyone), you still need to get some sort of exercise to keep your body functioning at top efficiency.

So you have disabilities or you just plain old have never worked out a day in your life. You simply need to find your starting point.

Easy, Take it slow, find out level you are starting out at. DO NOT injure yourself as this is NOT conducive to health.

Some of you may start out doing spin classes at the gym and some of you may start out learning how to get up off the floor unassisted.

Any time that you are working with restrictions and really don't have knowledge in how to exercise it is advisable to seek the advice of a personal trainer for a beginner routine and guidance on proper form as again to avoid injury.

In general for the beginner, Body weight circuits are the best bang for your buck (time) and if you listen to your body come with less fear of injury.

Body weight circuits get the whole body moving and motion is lotion.

The more you move the body the easier the body will move.

Just to name a few.

All of these can be done by any fitness level working within your current limits.

This means if you can only do 2 pushups…do 2 until you can do 3.

Actual workout routines will be published in another eBook.

It's going to be tough for you to break free from the stigma of "you are broken"

I get it, I was there once. Health and fitness is within the grasp of all and is achievable by all on different time lines only.

When you first start to exercise you may not have the knowledge or strength to keep the proper form to avoid injury.

With this said it is total ok to look to a chair for support when doing squats or lunges for example.

Remember it's not about being perfect!

Do what you can until you can do more.

You always want to get in a good routine with your exercise. At least 3 times a week, 4 or 5 would be better but never day after day.

Your body needs time to rest and repair and it's during these times that muscle growth occurs....NOT during the actual exercise.

Then of course the need for proper nutrition to fuel the machine that is your body.

You don't need to spend an hour at the gym. Including exercise in your plan doesn't mean you need to sign up for a gym or alter your schedule to include an hour of sweat time.

Don't try to do one-hour of nonstop exercise during the day; that can seem overwhelming, especially for beginners.

Instead, split it up into short mini-workouts, like a brisk walk outdoors after lunch and again before bed. Throw in some lunges during your walk or squats. It's well-documented that the benefits of exercise have a volume effect. As long as you get the same total amount of exercise during the day, that's just as effective.

So now.…what to expect as you start this new journey.

Your new found muscles are going to be sore, to the point you really want to quit.

DON'T.

Rest if you need for a day or 2 but get back on the horse.

You can feel moody.

You can feel lonely because you are going to be dedicated to you for awhile and that means some extra time away from friends (unless you can get them to workout also).

You and your health are not about how many pull ups or pushups you can do NOW or about how long you can do jumping jacks until you vomit.

It's about getting started. It's about teaching your body how to be fit and healthy again…It used to know and it will remember again but give it time. The people on these DVD's and infomercials have all been doing this for a long amount of time. Stop trying to keep up! Do what you can for now. Then when the time has come...you will be able to keep up with them and move on to the next level, if you are so inclined.

Do yourself a huge favor. Forget your ego....if you can only do one push up then do one....one good one, until you can do 2 and so on. Give yourself time to adapt and get used to the new routine. NOW...I did not just say be lazy and quit just cause you wanna. Remember I said 110% effort and if right now that's 1 push up then that's what it is but give it the 110%.

Say this in your head every day - I fight for me, I win for me! FOR ME!

Goals

Got to have them!

However make your goals achievable. This will help you to not abandon ship!

Remember marathon not a sprint.

Rome was not built in a day.

I'm also not a big fan of the scale.

All of you know you cant weigh yourselves once a week and be happy...you gotta step on that damn thing 8 times a day like a miracle happened and you lost 100 lbs in 2 hours while watching Opra.....Not gonna happen!

I personally would rather you dealt with measurements or how your clothes fit.

This is progress!

When you jump on the scale all the time you just defeat yourself....stop doing that!

So, are you ready? Ready to take your life back.

If not now, when?

Will you suddenly have more time next week?

Will a miracle happen that allows you all you need to do what you have to do?

That would be cool but im not betting my money so....let's go!

www.ingramcontent.com/pod-product-compliance
Lightning Source LLC
Chambersburg PA
CBHW030546290526
45786CB00004B/1884